Rhabdomyolysis

Nervous System Complications

Jacob McClain

Disclaimer

The information in this book is not meant to be used as medical advice; rather, it is meant only for educational reasons. It is not meant to replace expert medical supervision or be used for diagnosis. It is recommended that you discuss any medical problem with a healthcare provider before using any information provided.

The publisher and the author disclaim any liability for any injury allegedly resulting from material found in this book.

Table of Contents

Introduction

Definition and Overview of Rhabdomyolysis

A pathological condition known as rhabdomyolysis is defined by the quick disintegration of skeletal muscle fibers that have been wounded or damaged, which releases harmful intracellular substances into the bloodstream. Numerous factors, such as trauma, ischemia, medications, poisons, metabolic problems, and more, can lead to this condition.

There are two categories of clinical characteristics associated with rhabdomyolysis: systemic and local features. Systemic symptoms include fever, malaise, nausea, vomiting, disorientation, and abrupt renal failure, whereas local symptoms include muscular soreness, tenderness, swelling, and bruising.

Acute kidney damage, electrolyte imbalances, disseminated intravascular coagulation, compartment syndrome, and nervous system issues like seizures, stroke, and peripheral neuropathy are just a few of the consequences that can result from rhabdomyolysis.

Diagnosis of rhabdomyolysis entails testing high levels of creatine kinase, myoglobin in serum, and other biomarkers. Preventing acute renal injury and maintaining appropriate fluid resuscitation are the goals of rhabdomyolysis treatment and management. Treatment for rhabdomyolysis should include correcting electrolyte imbalances, closely monitoring urine output, and other measures in addition to identifying and eliminating the underlying cause of the condition.

In conclusion, rhabdomyolysis is a complicated medical disorder that causes skeletal muscle fibers that have been damaged or wounded to dissolve quickly, releasing intracellular muscle components into the bloodstream and extracellular space. It can have a number of reasons and result in a number of consequences, including issues with the neurological system. In order to reduce the possibility of long-term harm and enhance patient outcomes, early diagnosis and timely treatment are essential.

- **Rhabdomyolysis overview**

Rapid disintegration of damaged or injured skeletal muscle fibers results in the release of intracellular muscle contents into the circulation and extracellular space, which is a dangerous and potentially fatal disorder known as rhabdomyolysis. Numerous factors, such as trauma, ischemia, medications, poisons, metabolic problems, and more, might result in this condition.

Rhabdomyolysis's clinical signs and symptoms are highly indiscriminate, and the underlying cause determines how the condition develops. Both local and systemic symptoms, as well as early and late consequences, are present in rabdomyolysis. Systemic symptoms include fever, malaise, nausea, disorientation, and abrupt renal failure, whereas local symptoms include muscle soreness, weakness, bruising, swelling, and tenderness.

rhabdomyolysis is frequently caused by injury, strain, muscular hypoxia, infections, metabolic and electrolyte imbalances, medications, poisons, and genetic flaws. The etiology of rhabdomyolysis can be determined with the aid of a thorough history, physical examination, and laboratory workup.

Preventing acute renal injury and maintaining appropriate fluid resuscitation are the two main objectives of rhabdomyolysis management. The first step in treating rhabdomyolysis is determining the underlying cause and eliminating it. treatment should involve regular exams, close monitoring of urine output, correction of electrolyte imbalances, appropriate hydration to promote end-organ perfusion, and continual assessment of breathing, circulation, and airway.

In conclusion, rhabdomyolysis is a complicated medical disorder that causes skeletal muscle fibers that have been damaged or wounded to dissolve quickly, releasing intracellular muscle components into the bloodstream and extracellular space. It can have a number of reasons and result in a number of consequences, including issues with the neurological system. In order to reduce the possibility of long-term harm and enhance patient outcomes, early diagnosis and timely treatment are essential.

- **Scope and Importance of Nervous System Complications**

The nervous system consequences associated with rhabdomyolysis are quite serious and consequential since they might have grave and even fatal consequences. Rapid skeletal muscle fiber breakdown, or rhabdomyolysis, is a condition commonly linked to neuromuscular illnesses. It can lead to a number of nervous system consequences, such as delirium, seizures, peripheral neuropathy, altered mental status, and stroke. The quality of life of those who are affected by these issues may be greatly impacted and may have long-term consequences.

Given the dangerous and sometimes fatal nature of rhabdomyolysis as a syndrome, as well as its correlation with neuromuscular diseases, it is imperative that patients with rhabdomyolysis be identified and treated for any potential nervous system complications. Furthermore, the systemic effects of rhabdomyolysis—including its propensity to damage the nervous system—are highlighted by its consequences, which include acute renal failure, metabolic problems, and disseminated intravascular coagulation.

Healthcare professionals must use extreme caution when monitoring and treating individuals with rhabdomyolysis, especially in light of the possibility of developing nervous system problems. Improving patient outcomes and reducing the effects of these consequences require early detection, appropriate diagnostic evaluation, and prompt action. Moreover, a thorough study of rhabdomyolysis and its possible neurological ramifications is necessary, as it is linked to both sporadic and hereditary/recurrent cases.

Essentially, the extent and significance of nervous system issues associated with rhabdomyolysis call for increased clinical awareness, aggressive management, and further study to improve our knowledge of and ability to treat these potentially life-threatening consequences.

Chapter 1: Understanding Rhabdomyolysis

A medical disorder known as rhabdomyolysis is defined by the quick breakdown of injured muscle tissue and the subsequent release of muscle components into the blood. Numerous factors, including trauma, physical strain, infections, inherited illnesses, and some drugs, can cause this. Numerous consequences, including disseminated intravascular coagulation, acute renal damage, and electrolyte abnormalities, can result from the illness. Fever, malaise, nausea, confusion, agitation, delirium, and tea-colored urine are among the systemic symptoms of rhabdomyolysis. Understanding the telltale signs and symptoms of rhabdomyolysis is essential because major complications can be avoided with prompt diagnosis and treatment. One of the main goals of treatment when rhabdomyolysis is suspected is to prevent severe renal injury. Physicians need to understand the typical causes, diagnosis, and available treatments for rhabdomyolysis.

Causes and Mechanisms of Rhabdomyolysis

A medical disorder known as rhabdomyolysis is characterized by the quick disintegration of skeletal muscle tissue, which lets harmful intracellular components leak into the blood. Rhabdomyolysis in nervous system issues can result from a variety of reasons and mechanisms, some of which are as follows:

1. Trauma: Rhabdomyolysis can result from trauma to the skeletal muscle, such as a crush injury.

2. Ischemia: Rhabdomyolysis can be brought on by ischemia circumstances like compartment syndrome, which reduce the oxygen supply to the muscle cells.

3. Drugs and toxins: A number of substances can cause rhabdomyolysis, such as alcohol, some

pharmaceuticals (such as cocaine, antipsychotics, and statins), and toxic agents.

4. Metabolic and electrolyte disorders: Rhabdomyolysis can arise as a result of diseases including hypothyroidism, diabetic ketoacidosis, and electrolyte imbalances.

5. illnesses: Rhabdomyolysis has been linked to bacterial and viral illnesses, including influenza.

6. Exercise: Excessive exercise can cause rhabdomyolysis and muscle breakdown, especially in those who are not trained.

Rhabdomyolysis is caused by mechanisms that compromise the integrity of skeletal muscle, allowing intracellular muscle components—such as myoglobin—to be released directly into the bloodstream. As a result, there may be a number of problems, including acute kidney damage from myoglobin-induced nephrotoxicity.

To summarize, a variety of conditions, such as trauma, ischemia, toxins, metabolic abnormalities, infections, and exertion, can result in rhabdomyolysis. Toxic intracellular components are released into the bloodstream as a result of the illness, and this might have major side effects, such as involvement of the nervous system. For prompt diagnosis and treatment of rhabdomyolysis in clinical practice, it is essential to comprehend the various origins and mechanisms of the condition.

Clinical Presentation and Diagnosis

Rhabdomyolysis is a disorder that causes the skeletal muscle tissue to break down quickly. It can present clinically with both local and systemic symptoms. Systemic symptoms could include fever, malaise, nausea, and confusion, while local symptoms might include muscle soreness, weakness, bruising, swelling, and tenderness. Additionally, rhabdomyolysis can lead to nervous system consequences such as agitation, confusion, and, in severe cases, acute renal failure, which can influence neurological function.

A combination of laboratory results and clinical symptoms are used to diagnose rhabdomyolysis. Clinically, myalgia, weakness, and myoglobinuria—which appears as tea-colored urine—are the three signs of rhabdomyolysis. Determining significantly increased serum creatine kinase (CK) levels and the presence of myoglobin in the urine (myoglobinuria) is the gold standard for laboratory diagnosis. Patients with rhabdomyolysis may also exhibit aberrant results from other laboratory tests, including those measuring liver function, electrolyte levels, and renal function.

In conclusion, rhabdomyolysis presents clinically as a mix of systemic and local symptoms, with possible nervous system side effects including delirium, agitation, and acute renal failure. The three symptoms, together with the increased CK and myoglobinuria found in the lab, are used to make the diagnosis. It is imperative to identify and treat rhabdomyolysis as soon as possible in order to avoid major side effects, such as those that could harm the neurological system.

Chapter 2: Nervous System Involvement in Rhabdomyolysis

When rhabdomyolysis affects the nervous system, it can cause a number of consequences, such as agitation, delirium, and, in extreme situations, acute renal failure, which can impair neurological function. Although the precise mechanisms underpinning the neurological system's involvement in rhabdomyolysis are still unclear, it is believed that they arise from the withdrawal of an exogenous dopamine agonist or from a blockade of the dopamine receptor in the central nervous system.

Rapid disintegration of damaged or injured muscle cells is known as rhabdomyolysis, a complex medical disorder that can result in a number of consequences, including disseminated intravascular coagulation, acute renal failure (ARF), and electrolyte imbalances. In addition, medicines, poisons, infections, muscular ischemia, metabolic and electrolyte imbalances, genetic abnormalities, prolonged bed rest, and temperature-induced states such as neuroleptic malignant syndrome can cause the condition.

To summarize, the involvement of the neurological system in rhabdomyolysis can lead to a variety of consequences, such as acute renal failure, psychosis, and agitation. Though the precise mechanisms behind neurological system involvement are still unclear, it is believed that either the withdrawal of an exogenous dopamine agonist or a blockade of dopamine receptors in the central nervous system is the cause. It is imperative to identify and treat rhabdomyolysis as soon as possible in order to avoid major side effects, such as those that impact the neurological system.

Pathophysiology of Nervous System Impact

Though the exact pathophysiology of the nervous system impact in rhabdomyolysis is unknown, it is believed to be connected to the intracellular release of toxic substances into the bloodstream, which can have systemic effects, including those on the nervous system. A pathological disease known as rhabdomyolysis is characterized by damage to skeletal muscle cells that results in the release of poisonous intracellular material. Direct myocyte injury or energy supply interruption is the last common process that results in muscle injury and necrosis. This pathway causes the release of hazardous intracellular substances, such as myoglobin, into the blood circulation.

Myoglobin and other metabolites can be released into the bloodstream and cause a number of problems, including acute renal damage. Particularly, myoglobin's direct toxic effects on renal tubules can result in kidney damage. This systemic action can have secondary effects on the neurological system, which can result in consequences including agitation and psychosis. It also carries the risk of acute renal injury.

It is still unclear what precise pathways cause rhabdomyolysis's effects on the neurological system. Nonetheless, it is evident that a major factor in the pathophysiology of rhabdomyolysis and its possible effects on the nervous system is the release of hazardous intracellular components, such as myoglobin. To completely comprehend the precise pathways via which rhabdomyolysis affects the neurological system, more research is required.

Chapter 3: Rhabdomyolysis-Induced Neuropathy

Slight peripheral neuropathy is an uncommon but documented side effect of severe rhabdomyolysis. In the setting of rhabdomyolysis, a number of processes have been postulated to explain the development of peripheral neuropathy. These include the release of toxic intracellular constituents, metabolic alterations, and the effects of toxic or metabolic stress on muscle tissue. Severe cases of rhabdomyolysis seem to have a higher incidence of peripheral neuropathy.

Electromyography and nerve conduction investigations can be used to establish the diagnosis of rhabdomyolysis-induced peripheral neuropathy; however, little is known about the prognosis and neuropathy recovery in rhabdomyolysis patients. Preventing serious consequences such as peripheral neuropathy requires early detection of rhabdomyolysis and timely care, which includes fluid resuscitation and correction of electrolyte imbalances.

In conclusion, peripheral neuropathy is an uncommon side effect of severe rhabdomyolysis that is believed to have multiple causes. Electromyography and nerve conduction investigations can be used to confirm the diagnosis. It is crucial to identify and treat rhabdomyolysis as soon as possible to avoid these and other dangerous consequences.

Peripheral Neuropathy in Rhabdomyolysis

An uncommon but documented side effect of severe rhabdomyolysis is peripheral neuropathy. This disease is typified by intracellular muscle component secretion into the bloodstream and muscle destruction. Numerous theories have been put forth to explain peripheral neuropathy, such as rhabdomyolysis brought on by immobilization, alcohol-induced direct neurologic abnormalities, and peripheral neuropathy linked to compartment syndrome. Patients should be informed that rhabdomyolysis is likely to result in neurological abnormalities if they have underlying metabolic problems, such as those caused by long-term alcoholism. Peripheral neuropathy can be confirmed by electromyography and nerve conduction investigations; healing is advised through physical therapy and rehabilitation.

In the context of rhabdomyolysis, peripheral neuropathy might manifest as mixed nerve dysfunction, motor neuropathy, or sensory neuropathy. While motor symptoms might take the form of weakness and muscle atrophy, sensory symptoms can include numbness, tingling, and discomfort. This complication's complicated etiology may include ischemia injury, the harmful consequences of myoglobin that has been released, and inflammatory processes. The goal of managing peripheral neuropathy in rhabdomyolysis is to treat the neuropathic pain and address the underlying cause, such as fluid resuscitation, to avoid kidney damage caused by myoglobin. In these situations, close observation for potential side effects, such as renal failure, is crucial.

Improving the prognosis of rhabdomyolysis-associated peripheral neuropathy requires early detection and management.

Central Nervous System Involvement

Muscle necrosis and the release of intracellular muscle components into the bloodstream are hallmarks of the complicated medical illness known as rhabdomyolysis. Although symptoms relating to muscles are the main association with rhabdomyolysis, the central nervous system (CNS) can also be affected. Though the precise cause of the CNS's participation in rhabdomyolysis is unknown, it is believed to be the consequence of either the withdrawal of an exogenous drug or a dopamine receptor blockade in the central nervous system. Confusion, seizures, and coma are among the symptoms of central nervous system involvement that are more frequently observed in patients with acute renal injury and severe rhabdomyolysis. To avoid CNS consequences, rhabdomyolysis must be identified early and treated quickly. The underlying cause of the condition, such as fluid resuscitation to avoid myoglobin-induced kidney damage and symptomatic treatment for seizures and other neurological symptoms, are key components of treating CNS involvement in rhabdomyolysis. In these situations, close observation for potential side effects, such as renal failure, is crucial.

The CNS's involvement in rhabdomyolysis may be attributed to other reasons, in addition to the previously stated pathways. For instance, CNS symptoms may be brought on by electrolyte abnormalities such as hyponatremia and hyperkalemia. Furthermore, cerebral edema and elevated intracranial pressure can develop from metabolic acidosis brought on by rhabdomyolysis, both of which can induce neurological symptoms. Rhabdomyolysis can cause a wide range of symptoms of CNS involvement, from moderate confusion to a potentially fatal coma. As a result, it's critical to keep a careful eye out for any indications of CNS involvement in patients with rhabdomyolysis and to act quickly if needed. Admission to an intensive care unit and the application of sophisticated life support techniques, such as mechanical breathing and hemodialysis, may be necessary for the treatment of CNS involvement in rhabdomyolysis. All things considered, CNS involvement in rhabdomyolysis is a dangerous complication that needs to be identified and treated right away to avoid long-term brain damage.

Chapter 4: Neurological Sequelae of Rhabdomyolysis

Severe muscular necrosis can have rare but well-documented neurological consequences, especially in the form of peripheral neuropathy. In the setting of rhabdomyolysis, a number of pathways have been postulated for the development of peripheral neuropathy. These include rhabdomyolysis generated by immobilization, alcohol-induced direct neurologic abnormalities, and peripheral neuropathy related to compartment syndrome. Patients should be informed that rhabdomyolysis is likely to result in neurological abnormalities if they have underlying metabolic problems, such as those caused by long-term alcoholism. When rhabdomyolysis is present, peripheral neuropathy can be diagnosed and verified with electromyography and nerve conduction investigations. Physical treatment and rehabilitation come after the underlying cause is addressed, usually with fluid resuscitation and electrolyte imbalance repair. Despite being an uncommon side effect of rhabdomyolysis, peripheral neuropathy must be identified early and treated appropriately to maximize patient outcomes.

Rhabdomyolysis can result in peripheral neuropathy as well as other neurological side effects, such as involvement of the central nervous system (CNS). Confusion, seizures, and coma are among the symptoms of central nervous system involvement that are more frequently observed in patients with acute renal injury and severe rhabdomyolysis. Though the precise cause of the CNS's participation in rhabdomyolysis is unknown, it is believed to be the consequence of either the withdrawal of an exogenous drug or a dopamine receptor blockade in the central nervous system. Other potential causes of CNS involvement in rhabdomyolysis include metabolic acidosis and electrolyte abnormalities, such as hyperkalemia and hyponatremia. Rhabdomyolysis can cause a wide range of symptoms of CNS involvement, from moderate confusion to a potentially fatal coma. As a result, it's critical to keep a careful eye out for any indications of CNS involvement in patients with rhabdomyolysis and to act quickly if needed. Admission to an intensive care unit and the application of sophisticated life support techniques, such as mechanical breathing and hemodialysis, may be necessary for the treatment of CNS involvement in rhabdomyolysis. In general, rhabdomyolysis's neurological aftereffects have dangerous consequences that need to be identified and treated right away to avoid long-term brain damage.

Encephalopathy and Cognitive Impairment

Rare but documented side effects of rhabdomyolysis, a disorder marked by muscular necrosis and the release of intracellular muscle components into the bloodstream, include encephalopathy and cognitive impairment. Though the precise cause of encephalopathy and cognitive impairment in rhabdomyolysis is unknown, it is believed to be the consequence of either the withdrawal of an exogenous drug or a dopamine receptor blockade in the central nervous system. Confusion, seizures, and coma are some of the symptoms of encephalopathy, whereas memory loss, trouble focusing and paying attention, and problems with executive function are signs of cognitive impairment. Rhabdomyolysis can cause encephalopathy and cognitive impairment that range greatly in severity, from moderate disorientation to a potentially fatal coma. As such, it's critical to keep a close eye out for any indications of encephalopathy and cognitive impairment in individuals suffering from rhabdomyolysis and to act quickly to treat them if needed. Advanced life support techniques, including mechanical breathing and hemodialysis, may be necessary for the treatment of encephalopathy and cognitive impairment associated with rhabdomyolysis, as well as admission to an intensive care unit. To avoid encephalopathy and cognitive impairment, rhabdomyolysis must be identified early and treated quickly.

Encephalopathy and cognitive impairment in the context of rhabdomyolysis can also be associated with metabolic disruptions, such as electrolyte abnormalities (e.g., hyponatremia, hyperkalemia) and metabolic acidosis, which can impact brain function. Treating the underlying cause of rhabdomyolysis-related encephalopathy and cognitive impairment cntails correcting electrolyte imbalances, resuscitating fluid to prevent myoglobin-induced kidney damage, and providing supportive care for the central nervous system. Furthermore, in these circumstances, thorough observation for any consequences, such as renal failure, is crucial. Improving the prognosis of encephalopathy and cognitive impairment linked to rhabdomyolysis requires early detection and care. Consequently, when treating patients with rhabdomyolysis, medical professionals should keep a close eye out for these neurological side effects, especially if there has been extensive muscle damage and recent kidney damage.

Seizures and Other Neurological Manifestations

Muscle necrosis and the release of intracellular muscle components into the bloodstream are symptoms of the illness known as rhabdomyolysis. Acute kidney damage (AKI) can result from seizures, particularly status epilepticus, which can induce rhabdomyolysis. Rhabdomyolysis can also result from illness, heat stroke, muscle trauma, and the intake of certain chemicals or drugs. Although the frequency of rhabdomyolysis in seizures is unclear, it appears that rhabdomyolysis incidence is correlated with the number and length of seizures. Urine that is dark brown in color and muscle weakness or soreness are early clinical signs of rhabdomyolysis caused by seizures. Life-threatening conditions such as severe electrolyte imbalances and AKI can result from rhabdomyolysis. Rhabdomyolysis is linked to a diverse range of neurological illnesses, the majority of which are connected with epilepsy.

chapter 5: Diagnostic Approaches

A combination of clinical examination, history, laboratory investigations, muscle biopsy, and genetic testing is used in the diagnosis of rhabdomyolysis. The primary diagnostic instruments and factors are as follows:

1. Clinical examination: Check for any evidence of muscular injury or damage, such as discomfort, weakness, or swelling.

An essential part of the diagnostic process for rhabdomyolysis is the clinical examination. The traditional trio of symptoms consists of myalgia, weakness, and dark urine, or myoglobinuria. Less than 10% of patients exhibit this triad; hence, a high index of suspicion is required, particularly in those with established risk factors such as trauma, sepsis, muscle illness, and immobilization. Even in patients who are non verbalizing, a neuromuscular examination that concentrates on the limbs can offer significant physical cues, such as an evaluation of color, pulse, feeling, muscle power, and size.

Furthermore, in individuals with rhabdomyolysis, the diagnostic diagnosis may be guided by the existence of involvement in other organ systems. As a result, early identification and diagnosis of rhabdomyolysis depend on a thorough clinical examination and a patient history.

2. History: Determine the existence of any possible risk factors, including immobilization, trauma, infection, and muscular diseases.

A comprehensive medical history can be used to determine possible risk factors and offer hints about the underlying cause of muscle injury. Important facets of the past to take into account are:

i. Recent trauma or injury: Rhabdomyolysis can result from trauma, including crush injuries.

ii. Prolonged immobilization: Rhabdomyolysis and muscle damage can also result from prolonged immobilization, such as bed rest or cast immobilization.

iii. Presence of additional risk factors: Respiratory distress, muscle illness, and the use of specific drugs are among the additional risk factors that can raise the risk of rhabdomyolysis.

iv. Muscular discomfort or weakness: Individuals may experience this condition, which may indicate rhabdomyolysis early on.

v. Other organ system involvement: Patients with rhabdomyolysis may benefit from guidance in their diagnostic diagnosis if they have other organ system involvement, such as cardiomyopathies, endocrinopathies, or encephalopathies.

In order to diagnose, evaluate, and treat rhabdomyolysis, medical personnel can gain a deeper understanding of the patient's risk factors and possible underlying causes by obtaining a thorough history.

3. Laboratory studies: Serum creatine kinase (CK) levels: The most sensitive and dependable marker of muscle damage is elevated CK levels.

Myoglobin levels in urine: myoglobinuria may be indicated by dark brown urine.
Other blood enzymes: Rhabdomyolysis may also result in high levels of other enzymes, including lactate dehydrogenase (LDH) and aspartate aminotransferase (AST).

An integral part of the diagnostic strategy for rhabdomyolysis is laboratory research. An increased serum creatine kinase (CK) level is the most reliable and sensitive marker of muscle injury. The following additional lab tests could be helpful in the diagnosis of rhabdomyolysis:

i. Urine myoglobin levels: myoglobinuria, a defining feature of rhabdomyolysis, may be indicated by dark brown urine.

ii. Serum enzymes: Rhabdomyolysis may also result in high levels of other enzymes, including lactate dehydrogenase (LDH) and aspartate aminotransferase (AST).

iii. Complete blood count (CBC): CBC can be used to detect anemia or thrombocytopenia, two possible rhabdomyolysis complications.

iv. Serum chemistries: Serum chemistries, such as liver function tests (LFTs), creatinine, glucose, calcium, potassium, phosphate, uric acid, and blood urea nitrogen (BUN), can assist in identifying possible rhabdomyolysis consequences, such as acute kidney damage (AKI).

v. Prothrombin time (PT): PT can be used to detect coagulopathy and other possible rhabdomyolysis side effects.

vi. Muscle biopsy: A muscle biopsy can help determine the underlying cause of rhabdomyolysis and offer histological proof of muscle damage.

When individuals with rhabdomyolysis also have involvement in other organ systems, the combination of these conditions may aid in directing the diagnostic assessment. Usually, a coherent history and an increased CK level are enough to support the diagnosis of rhabdomyolysis

4. Muscle biopsy: A muscle biopsy can help determine the underlying cause of rhabdomyolysis and offer histological evidence of muscle damage.

When treating patients who may have rhabdomyolysis or other metabolic myopathies, a muscle biopsy is a crucial diagnostic procedure. When rhabdomyolysis is present, the time of the muscle biopsy is crucial. Generally speaking, diagnostic muscle biopsies should be postponed for at least one month, if not longer. Glycolytic enzyme tests and enzyme immunohistochemistry are examined in muscle biopsies to diagnose rhabdomyolysis. A muscle biopsy can help determine the underlying cause of rhabdomyolysis and offer histological proof of muscle damage. A muscle biopsy, however, is frequently unhelpful in the context of acute rhabdomyolysis since it usually shows extensive muscle fiber necrosis, irrespective of the underlying cause (e.g., exertional, traumatic, toxic, or genetic). Consequently, patients with suspected myopathy who are unable to receive a genetic test diagnosis are typically the ones who undergo a muscle biopsy. A muscle biopsy may be considered in rhabdomyolysis patients if other diagnostic tests are unsatisfactory or if there is a strong suspicion of an underlying myopathy. A muscle biopsy is an important diagnostic tool for evaluating rhabdomyolysis overall, but it should only be done sparingly and in combination with other procedures.

5. Genetic testing: Genetic testing may be taken into consideration to discover potential genetic diseases in situations where an acquired or

intrinsic cause of rhabdomyolysis cannot be readily determined.

In order to distinguish between acquired and inherited causes of rhabdomyolysis, genetic testing is a crucial part of the diagnostic process. Disorders of mitochondrial oxidative phosphorylation, fatty acid beta-oxidation, and glycogen metabolism can all lead to an inherited propensity for rhabdomyolysis. Certain genetic abnormalities linked to rhabdomyolysis, such as impairment in carnitine palmitoyltransferase II (CPT-II), can be identified through genetic testing.

Gene panels and/or whole exome sequencing may be considered in patients with recurrent rhabdomyolysis who do not have a specific clinical characteristic or a known acquired cause. It is anticipated that new genetic variables that predispose people to recurrent rhabdomyolysis will be discovered as clinical genetic testing and whole exome sequencing become more generally accessible.

To sum up, genetic testing is an important diagnostic technique for rhabdomyolysis since it can help uncover particular genetic flaws linked to the disorder and provide guidance for individuals who experience recurrent episodes of rhabdomyolysis.

6. Imaging studies: Although radiography, CT, and MRI are generally not helpful in the initial diagnosis of rhabdomyolysis, they could be required in some situations, including when a patient needs a head CT scan for head trauma or seizure activity or when fractures are suspected.

The degree of muscle involvement, complications like myonecrosis and muscular atrophy, and other etiologies or concurrent injuries causing musculoskeletal swelling and pain can all be assessed with the help of imaging studies, though they are not usually the primary diagnostic tool for rhabdomyolysis. The underlying etiology of rhabdomyolysis will determine the imaging results, although, generally speaking, the muscles will show symptoms of edema and/or hemorrhage. When diagnosing underlying bone fractures, joint dislocations, and occasionally soft tissue edema, computed tomography (CT) is helpful. When fasciotomy is being investigated as a therapeutic option, magnetic resonance imaging (MRI) is the preferred technique for assessing the distribution and extension of the afflicted muscles. Additionally, MRI can be used to distinguish rhabdomyolysis from other diseases such as compartment syndrome, which typically result in the destruction or displacement of normal muscle fibers. All rhabdomyolysis patients exhibited diffusely mild-to-prominent-degree involvement of the anterior thigh muscles on fluid-sensitive sequences. Assessing the degree of muscle involvement in rhabdomyolysis can also be done with ultrasound. In summary, imaging techniques can be helpful in determining the degree of muscle involvement and finding underlying bone fractures or dislocations, even if they are not usually utilized as the primary diagnostic tool for rhabdomyolysis. The best method to assess the distribution and extension of the impacted muscles is magnetic resonance imaging (MRI).

When individuals with rhabdomyolysis also have involvement in other organ systems, the combination of these conditions may aid in directing the diagnostic assessment. Muscle biopsies or other testing may not be required following a single incident of rhabdomyolysis if no acquired cause is found, unless there is additional evidence or repeated episodes.

Imaging Techniques for Nervous System Complications

A variety of imaging modalities can be employed to assess nervous system problems associated with rhabdomyolysis. The primary method for assessing peripheral neuropathy in rhabdomyolysis patients is magnetic resonance imaging (MRI). Aside from determining the degree of muscle involvement, MRI can also be utilized to spot underlying bone fractures or dislocations. Joint dislocation, underlying bone fractures, and occasionally soft tissue edema can all be detected with computed tomography (CT) scans. Assessing the degree of muscle involvement in rhabdomyolysis can also be done with ultrasound. It's crucial to remember, nevertheless, that imaging tests are usually employed to determine the degree of muscle involvement and spot underlying bone fractures or dislocations rather than as the main diagnostic method for rhabdomyolysis. In general, imaging methods are not usually employed as the main diagnostic approach for rhabdomyolysis, even if they can be helpful in assessing nervous system issues.

Laboratory and Neurophysiological Assessments

Laboratory and neurophysiological tests can be used to identify nervous system problems in rhabdomyolysis. The most sensitive laboratory test for determining the kind of muscular injury that might result in rhabdomyolysis is creatine kinase (CK), which is frequently used in the diagnosis of rhabdomyolysis. Furthermore, even in patients who are nonverbal, a neuromuscular examination that concentrates on the limbs can offer crucial physical cues, such as an evaluation of color, pulse, feeling, muscle power, and size.

In certain instances, additional workup—such as muscle biopsies, genetic testing, and electrodiagnostic studies—may be necessary to assess probable nervous system problems and underlying myopathies. While muscle biopsy and genetic tests can be utilized to uncover underlying muscle illnesses or genetic problems linked to rhabdomyolysis, electrodiagnostic examinations can aid in evaluating the function of the nerves and muscles.

Overall, the examination of nervous system problems in rhabdomyolysis can benefit from a thorough approach that includes laboratory assessments and, where necessary, neurophysiological testing, particularly in cases where an underlying myopathy is suspected.

Chapter 6: Clinical Management

A multidisciplinary strategy is used in the clinical therapy of rhabdomyolysis with nervous system consequences. The major goals of this approach are to prevent acute kidney damage (AKI), maintain appropriate fluid resuscitation, and resolve electrolyte imbalances. Preventing problems and guaranteeing the best possible outcome for the patient are the main objectives. Important facets of clinical management consist of:

1. Assessment of ABCs: Monitoring respiratory, circulatory, and airway function is essential for treating rhabdomyolysis.

2. Identification and correction of the inciting cause: Effective management of rhabdomyolysis requires the identification and treatment of the underlying cause.

3. Fluid resuscitation: To enhance end-organ perfusion and avoid AKI, adequate fluid resuscitation is required.

4. Electrolyte management: The management of rhabdomyolysis requires careful observation and correction of electrolyte abnormalities, such as those involving potassium and phosphate.

5. Renal support: Using diuretics, hemodialysis, or continuous renal replacement treatment may be required in situations of AKI.

6. Neurological monitoring: The management of rhabdomyolysis with consequences for the nervous system requires close monitoring of neurological function, particularly muscle strength and sensation.

7. Treatment of underlying problems: In order to effectively manage rhabdomyolysis, it is imperative to address any underlying conditions, such as infections or metabolic disorders.

8. Supportive care: Giving the patient the right kind of support, like physical therapy and pain management, can help them get better overall.

In conclusion, a multidisciplinary approach is required for the clinical therapy of rhabdomyolysis with nervous system consequences. This approach centers on maintaining appropriate fluid resuscitation, avoiding acute renal injury, treating electrolyte imbalances, and constantly monitoring neurological function.

Treatment Strategies for Rhabdomyolysis

Treatment for rhabdomyolysis with consequences for the nervous system entails a multidisciplinary approach with the goals of minimizing acute kidney damage (AKI), treating electrolyte imbalances, and maintaining appropriate fluid resuscitation. Key components of treatment plans for rhabdomyolysis with consequences for the neurological system include the following:

- Fluid Resuscitation: To enhance end-organ perfusion and avoid AKI, adequate fluid resuscitation is necessary. The key to preventing renal damage and renal failure is early intervention along with vigorous hydration.

- Electrolyte Management: Handling rhabdomyolysis requires careful observation and treatment of electrolyte abnormalities, such as those involving potassium and phosphate.

- Renal Support: Continuous renal replacement therapy, hemodialysis, or the use of diuretics may all be required in cases of AKI.

- Identifying and Treating the Underlying Cause: As part of the treatment plan, it's critical to determine and treat the underlying cause of rhabdomyolysis, such as trauma, infection, or toxins.

- Neurological Monitoring: In order to manage rhabdomyolysis with nervous system problems, it is imperative to closely assess neurological function, particularly muscle strength and sensation.

- Prevention: Efforts should be taken to prevent rhabdomyolysis whenever an avoidable inciting cause has been found. For instance, if exercise is causing or aggravating rhabdomyolysis, it should be minimized or avoided.

- Supportive Care: Improving the patient's overall result can be achieved by providing suitable supportive care, such as physical therapy and pain management.

Dialysis may be required if kidney damage and acute renal failure have already begun in severe cases, and drugs like bicarbonate and specific types of diuretics may be administered to help manage the condition. The general care of rhabdomyolysis also includes home remedies and preventive measures, such as drinking enough water and seeing a doctor when feeling ill. Treatment for rhabdomyolysis with complications to the nervous system generally entails a multidisciplinary approach with an emphasis on keeping fluid resuscitation adequate, avoiding AKI, treating electrolyte imbalances, and continuously monitoring neurological function.

Interventions for Nervous System Complications

A multidisciplinary strategy for treating nervous system consequences in rhabdomyolysis is necessary. This approach should address electrolyte imbalances, prevent acute kidney damage (AKI), maintain appropriate fluid resuscitation, and address the underlying cause. To control nervous system issues, specialized therapies could be required in addition to these general therapy options. For instance, physical therapy and occupational therapy may be suggested to increase muscular strength and function if peripheral neuropathy is present. In order to release pressure on the impacted muscles, a fasciotomy might be required if compartment syndrome is present. Antiepileptic drugs may be administered to treat seizures in cases of rhabdomyolysis with central nervous system involvement, such as encephalopathy or seizures, and supportive care may be required to treat additional neurological symptoms.

All things considered, treating nervous system issues in rhabdomyolysis necessitates a thorough strategy that takes care of electrolyte imbalances, maintains appropriate fluid resuscitation, and addresses the underlying cause. Nervous system issues may require specific interventions, and a multidisciplinary team approach is frequently required to guarantee the best possible outcome for the patient.

Chapter 7: Rehabilitation and Long-Term Outcomes

The severity of the ailment and the underlying cause of rhabdomyolysis determine rehabilitation and long-term results. Patients with rhabdomyolysis typically require many months to regain muscle mass, and some may continue to feel pain for a few years after the injury. Rhabdomyolysis rehabilitation techniques usually entail a multidisciplinary approach with an emphasis on function restoration, muscle strength restoration, and problem avoidance. In rhabdomyolysis, important elements of recovery and long-term results include:

1. Physical therapy: Physical therapy aids in increasing range of motion, flexibility, and muscle strength. Exercises like stretching, strengthening, and agility training may be part of this.

2. Occupational therapy: Occupational therapy helps increase safety in daily tasks and assists patients with rhabdomyolysis in regaining their

independence. Training in jobs, recreation, and self-care may be part of this.

3. Risk stratification: To stop further bouts of recurrent rhabdomyolysis, risk stratification is crucial. This could entail figuring out and treating underlying issues, such as a protracted healing process or certain triggers.

4. Return to sport: A gradual return to sports or physical activity may be required in situations of exertional rhabdomyolysis. To stop recurring occurrences, fitness practitioners need to comprehend the significance of starting at a baseline fitness level and providing progressive training.

5. Long-term follow-up: To secure the best possible outcome for the patient and to keep an eye out for any issues, long-term follow-up is essential.

Overall, a multidisciplinary strategy centered on regaining muscle strength, enhancing function, and averting problems is necessary for rehabilitation and long-term results in rhabdomyolysis patients. Long-term follow-up and close observation are necessary to provide the best potential outcome for the patient.

Rehabilitation Approaches for Neurological Recovery

Strategies for neurological recovery during rehabilitation are essential for rhabdomyolysis patients in order to improve mobility, restore muscular function, and avoid problems. For an individual to progress in independence, safety, and confidence, the transitions from acute care to inpatient and outpatient rehabilitation settings must be coordinated. The following are essential elements of rhabdomyolysis rehabilitation strategies for neurological recovery:

1. Physical Therapy: Enhancing muscle strength, flexibility, and range of motion requires physical therapy. It usually consists of range-of-motion exercises as part of a contracture prevention

program, then aerobic training and gradually increasing resistance training.

2. Occupational Therapy: The goal of occupational therapy is to assist people in regaining their independence in everyday living, employment, and pleasure. In order to increase safety and quality of life, it may involve training in self-care, work-related tasks, and adaptive techniques.

3. Prevention of Overexertion: To stop additional muscle deterioration during rehabilitation, it's critical to avoid overexertion. To help clients recover, fitness experts and therapists must recognize the value of the client's starting fitness level and offer progressive training.

4. Long-Term Follow-Up: To evaluate healing, treat any lingering symptoms, and stop further bouts of rhabdomyolysis, long-term observation and follow-up are crucial.

In conclusion, physical and occupational therapy are key components of rehabilitation strategies for neurological recovery in rhabdomyolysis, as they help to promote independence and restore muscular function. Ensuring long-term follow-up and avoiding overexertion are two other critical components of the rehabilitation process.

Long-Term Impact on Nervous System Function

Rapid disintegration of damaged or injured muscle tissue results in the release of toxic intracellular material into the circulatory system, which is a significant medical disorder known as rhabdomyolysis. Numerous issues, including disseminated intravascular coagulation, acute renal failure (ARF), and electrolyte abnormalities, may result from this. Rhabdomyolysis can cause peripheral neuropathy, which can have a substantial long-term effect on nervous system function.

One uncommon side effect of rhabdomyolysis is peripheral neuropathy, which can be brought on by long-term alcohol consumption-related metabolic alterations. In the hands and feet, this complication may include tingling, numbness, and muscle weakness. Although the precise processes by which rhabdomyolysis causes peripheral neuropathy are not entirely understood, it is thought to be connected to the poisonous compounds that are released from injured muscle tissue.

In summary, peripheral neuropathy, which can result in tingling, numbness, and muscle weakness in the hands and feet, can have a long-term negative influence on the functioning of the nervous system in rhabdomyolysis patients. Long-term alcohol consumption can make this problem worse. It is thought to be associated with the release of poisonous chemicals from injured muscle tissue.

Chapter 8: Prevention Strategies

Serious medical conditions, such as disseminated intravascular coagulation, acute renal failure, and electrolyte abnormalities, can result from rhabdomyolysis. Due to the possibility of peripheral neuropathy, rhabdomyolysis can have a substantial long-term effect on nervous system function. A rare side effect of rhabdomyolysis is peripheral neuropathy, which can include tingling, numbness, and weakness in the hands and feet. In order to avoid rhabdomyolysis, one should:

1. Acclimate to heat and levels of physical activity prior to extended durations of work: This can assist the body in adjusting to the demands of physical exercise and lower the risk of rhabdomyolysis.

2. Remain hydrated: Getting adequate water and other fluids will help you stay hydrated and avoid dehydration, both of which can lead to rhabdomyolysis.

3. Take breaks in a cooler area. The body can recuperate from heat shock, and the danger of rhabdomyolysis can be decreased by taking regular rests in a cooler setting.

4. Learn the symptoms and indicators of illnesses brought on by the heat: By being aware of the early warning signals of heat-related disorders, people can avoid rhabdomyolysis and seek medical assistance as soon as possible.

5. Start an exercise regimen gradually and give yourself enough time off. Rhabdomyolysis can be avoided by introducing an exercise regimen gradually and giving the body time to heal.

6. Avoid extreme dehydration and overheating. Rhabdomyolysis can be caused by these conditions; therefore, it's critical to maintain a good balance between physical activity and rest.

7. Assess medical advice prior to starting any new, intense physical activity: A medical expert can offer specific recommendations and

directions on safe physical activity practices that lower the danger of rhabdomyolysis.

People can lessen their chance of acquiring rhabdomyolysis and the issues related to the nervous system by implementing these preventative techniques.

Identifying High-Risk Populations

Although everyone is susceptible to rabdomyolysis, some groups are more vulnerable than others. Among the high-risk categories are:

1. Occupational Risk: Individuals who do physically demanding jobs or labor in hot conditions are more vulnerable. This includes first responders, police officers, firefighters (both structural and wildland), farm and construction workers, forgers, and active-duty military personnel.

2. Sportsmen and Physically Demanding Employment: People who work in physically demanding occupations requiring a lot of physical effort, together with athletes, are more likely to develop rhabdomyolysis.

3. Traumatic Injuries and Exertional Factors: People who participate in high-intensity or prolonged activities, as well as those who are engaged in activities that may result in traumatic injuries, are also more susceptible.

4. Substance Use and Diseases: Risk factors for rhabdomyolysis include taking illegal drugs, drinking too much alcohol, and having certain diseases (such as the flu, HIV, salmonella, staph, strep, and Epstein-Barr virus).

5. Genetic abnormalities: Rhabdomyolysis can also be caused by underlying genetic abnormalities, which raises the risk for those who are impacted.

It's crucial to remember that rhabdomyolysis can strike anybody at any degree of fitness; even highly fit people, like firefighters and sportsmen, can have it. Thus, controlling and preventing rhabdomyolysis requires early symptom detection and knowledge of the risk factors.

Preventive Measures for Rhabdomyolysis-Related Nervous System Complications

The following are preventive steps for nervous system issues associated with rhabdomyolysis:

1. Hydration and Heat Avoidance: Reducing the likelihood of related nervous system problems can be achieved by preventing rhabdomyolysis through proper hydration and heat avoidance.

2. Early Treatment: Life-threatening consequences, especially those affecting the neurological system, can be avoided by treating rhabdomyolysis as soon as possible.

3. Identifying High-Risk Populations: Preventive measures can be put into place by identifying people who are more likely to experience rhabdomyolysis, such as athletes or those in physically demanding occupations.

4. Treatment of Underlying Causes: Rehabdomyolysis's associated problems, particularly nervous system-related ones, can be avoided by treating its underlying causes, which include trauma, infections, and substance abuse.

The likelihood of developing rhabdomyolysis and its possible effects on the neurological system can be decreased by putting these preventive measures into practice.

Chapter 9: Case Studies

Case Studies in Rhabdomyolysis: Complications for the Nervous System

1. Cocaine-Induced Rhabdomyolysis: According to a case study, a patient used cocaine and developed rhabdomyolysis, which resulted in peripheral neuropathy. The patient complained of tingling in the hands and feet, numbness, and weakening in the muscles. With an emphasis on aggressive fluid resuscitation and treating the underlying cause, the patient's prognosis was deemed to be good.

2. Rhabdomyolysis in a Firefighter: Following their entrapment in a flaming building, a firefighter had rhabdomyolysis, which resulted in severe kidney damage and compartment syndrome. The patient experienced muscle weakness, edema, and excruciating agony. Treatment for compartment syndrome included supportive care for renal damage, rapid fluid resuscitation, and surgery.

3. Rhabdomyolysis in a Marathon Runner: Following the completion of a long-distance race, a marathon runner had rhabdomyolysis, which resulted in severe renal damage and electrolyte imbalances. Among the patient's symptoms were black urine, weakness, and cramping in the muscles. For renal injury, treatment included electrolyte replacement, rapid fluid resuscitation, and supportive care.

These case examples emphasize the significance of diagnosing and treating rhabdomyolysis as soon as possible in order to avoid potentially fatal consequences, such as those that impact the neurological system.

Real-life Cases Illustrating Nervous System Complications

Numerous real-world instances have demonstrated how rhabdomyolysis can cause nervous system issues. Peripheral neuropathy, injury to the peripheral nerves, and other neurological disorders are some of these consequences. For example, a case study described a patient who developed peripheral neuropathy, an uncommon side effect of rhabdomyolysis, along with tingling, numbness, and muscle weakness in the hands and feet. Four patients with drug-induced rhabdomyolysis were reported in another investigation to have peripheral nerve injuries, three of whom were unconscious and one of whom was lethargic. These cases highlight how critical it is to identify and treat nervous system issues when rhabdomyolysis is present. For the entire care and treatment of people with rhabdomyolysis, early detection and control of these consequences are essential.

Lessons Learned and Best Practices

Rhabdomyolysis can result in a number of issues, including nervous system-related ones. It is typified by the disintegration of muscle tissue and the release of intracellular components into the circulatory system. The literature has yielded a number of important takeaways and recommended practices, including:

1. Early Recognition and Diagnosis: Although rhabdomyolysis has distinctive clinical, biochemical, and radiologic characteristics, a high index of suspicion is necessary for an accurate diagnosis in a timely manner. The various causes of rhabdomyolysis, such as muscle strain, illegal drug usage, alcohol misuse, prescription drugs, trauma, and immobility, should be known to medical professionals.

2. Vigorous Fluid Resuscitation: Vigorous fluid resuscitation is the cornerstone of treatment for rhabdomyolysis. Hydration must be aggressively and promptly maintained to avoid severe renal failure and other systemic consequences.

3. The identification and management of the underlying causes of rhabdomyolysis are of utmost importance. Treating severe injuries, substance misuse, or other contributing factors

may be necessary in order to stop more muscle damage and related consequences.

4. Prevention of Complications: Medical professionals need to be on the lookout for potential rhabdomyolysis side effects, including acidosis, disseminated intravascular coagulation, acute renal damage, arrhythmias, and clcctrolytc abnormalities. Proactive management and early identification of these consequences are essential.

5. Supportive Care and Monitoring: Individuals with rhabdomyolysis need to be closely watched, get supportive care, and have their breathing, circulation, and airway constantly assessed. Frequent exams and the correction of electrolyte imbalances are crucial elements of care.

Healthcare providers can enhance the early detection, treatment, and avoidance of nervous system issues linked to rhabdomyolysis by implementing these lessons and best practices into clinical care.

Chapter 10: Future Directions in Research

A complicated medical disorder called rhabdomyolysis can have a number of side effects, including nervous system damage. There is still much to learn about the pathophysiology, diagnosis, and therapy of rhabdomyolysis, despite tremendous advancements in these areas. Future research initiatives include the following:

1. "Molecular Mechanisms of Kidney Injury Induced by Rhabdomyolysis": Understanding the molecular pathways behind kidney impairment caused by rhabdomyolysis has been the focus of recent research. New treatments and preventive measures may be developed as a result of more research in this field.

2. Identification of Novel Biomarkers: Early diagnosis and condition monitoring may be aided by the discovery of novel biomarkers for rhabdomyolysis. More sensitive and accurate diagnostic tests may result from research in this field.

3. Prevention Strategies: More investigation is required to find practical rhabdomyolysis prevention measures, especially for high-risk

groups like sportsmen and military personnel. This can entail looking at the importance of staying hydrated, avoiding the heat, and taking other precautions.

4. Management of Nervous System Complications: Additional study is required to identify the underlying causes of nervous system complications in rhabdomyolysis and to create efficient therapies for these issues.

Researchers can enhance the care and results of people with rhabdomyolysis and its related consequences by carrying out more studies on the pathogenesis, diagnosis, and treatment of this disorder.

Current Trends in Rhabdomyolysis Research

Recent studies on rhabdomyolysis have concentrated on a number of topics, such as the condition's prevalence and trends, the molecular mechanisms behind kidney damage brought on by rhabdomyolysis, and the condition's clinical signs and diagnosis. Among the most recent developments in rhabdomyolysis research are:

1. Increase in Exertional Rhabdomyolysis Incidence: According to a study, between 2011 and 2014, the frequency of exertional rhabdomyolysis quadrupled. This pattern emphasizes the need for additional study, especially in high-risk groups, to determine the causes and preventative measures for rhabdomyolysis.

2. Molecular Mechanisms of Kidney Injury Induced by Rhabdomyolysis: Understanding the molecular pathways behind kidney impairment caused by rhabdomyolysis has been the focus of recent research. The results of this study may guide the creation of fresh remedies and prophylactic measures.

3. Rhabdomyolysis Clinical Manifestations and Diagnosis: Enhancing rhabdomyolysis's clinical signs and diagnosis has also been the target of

research. This entails finding new biomarkers and enhancing diagnostic procedures to help in the early detection and management of the illness.

4. Prevention Strategies: More study is required to determine the best ways to avoid rhabdomyolysis, especially in high-risk groups like athletes and military personnel. This can entail looking at the importance of staying hydrated, avoiding the heat, and taking other precautions.

Researchers can enhance the care and results of people with rhabdomyolysis by carrying out more studies on the etiology, diagnosis, and therapy of this illness.

Conclusion

To sum up, rhabdomyolysis is a complicated illness that can cause a number of side effects, including nervous system problems. The cornerstone of treatment for rhabdomyolysis is intensive fluid resuscitation, and the prognosis is generally regarded as good. Arrhythmias, electrolyte imbalances, acute renal damage, acidosis, volume depletion, compartment syndrome, and disseminated intravascular coagulation are just a few of the consequences that the disorder can cause. In order to further rhabdomyolysis research and clinical practice, it is imperative that:

1. Promote early identification and diagnosis since rhabdomyolysis has distinctive radiologic, clinical, and laboratory characteristics that call for a high degree of suspicion in order to be diagnosed in a timely manner.

2. Determine the underlying causes to stop additional muscle loss and related consequences. This may entail treating traumatic injuries, substance addiction, or other contributing factors.

3. Avoid acute renal damage, as this is a frequent side effect of rhabdomyolysis.

4. Look into the molecular mechanisms of kidney damage caused by rhabdomyolysis; this

may help with the creation of fresh remedies and prophylactic measures.

5. Enhance rhabdomyolysis's clinical signs and diagnosis, including the discovery of new biomarkers and the advancement of diagnostic procedures.

Healthcare providers can improve the care and results of patients with rhabdomyolysis and the nervous system problems it causes by attending to these factors.

- Recapitulation of Key Findings

Rhabdomyolysis is a neurological condition that affects a wide range of neurological entities. Its prevalence and clinical spectrum are varied, and most cases have a fair prognosis with very few serious complications. Rhabdomyolysis, which has several etiologies, non-specific symptoms, and systemic consequences that make diagnosis difficult, continues to be a significant clinical challenge. Vigorous fluid resuscitation is the cornerstone of treatment for rhabdomyolysis, and although the prognosis varies greatly and depends on the underlying etiologies and comorbidities, it is typically regarded as good. Acute renal damage and compartment syndrome are possible side effects of rhabdomyolysis. In order to help with the early identification and treatment of rhabdomyolysis, research has concentrated on enhancing the condition's clinical signs, diagnosis, and prognostic factors.

- Implications for Clinical Practice and Research

There are important ramifications for rhabdomyolysis research and clinical practice, especially with regard to nervous system problems. The diagnosis of rhabdomyolysis can be difficult because of its non-specific symptoms, various etiologies, and systemic consequences. Nonetheless, the outlook is usually favorable, and the mainstay of care is aggressive fluid resuscitation. Enhancing early recognition and diagnosis, determining underlying causes, and preventing acute renal injury—a major result of rhabdomyolysis—are all critical to improving clinical practice. Understanding the molecular mechanisms behind kidney damage caused by rhabdomyolysis, refining the clinical presentation and diagnosis of the condition, and devising practical preventative measures—especially for high-risk individuals—should be the main goals of this field of study. Healthcare providers can improve the care and results of patients with rhabdomyolysis and the nervous system problems it causes by attending to these factors.

References

Adnet, F., Baud, F. J., & Vicaut, E. (2001). Rhabdomyolysis in the emergency department: 26 cases. European Journal of Emergency Medicine, 8(1), 3-7.

Better, O. S., & Stein, J. H. (1990). Early management of shock and prophylaxis of acute renal failure in traumatic rhabdomyolysis. New England Journal of Medicine, 322(12), 825-829.

Bosch, X., Poch, E., & Grau, J. M. (2009). Rhabdomyolysis and acute kidney injury. New England Journal of Medicine, 361(1), 62-72. https://journals.cambridgemedia.com.au/applicat ion/files/8116/0792/5332/choy.pdf

Choy, K. W., Wong, W. S., & Chan, T. M. (2014). Rhabdomyolysis cases and acute kidney injury: A 10-year retrospective review at a tertiary hospital in Hong Kong. Hong Kong Journal of Emergency Medicine, 21(2), 87-94. https://medscidiscovery.com/index.php/msd/artic le/view/133

Huerta-Alardín, A. L., Varon, J., & Marik, P. E. (2015). Bench-to-bedside review: Rhabdomyolysis – An overview for clinicians. Critical Care, 19(1), 1-10. https://www.ncbi.nlm.nih.gov/pmc/articles/PMC 4365849/

Kaur, R., & Kaur, H. (2021). A rare complication of rhabdomyolysis: Peripheral neuropathy. Cureus, 13(3), e14022. https://www.cureus.com/articles/46125-a-rare-complication-of-rhabdomyolysis-peripheral-neuropathy

Melli, G., Chaudhry, V., Cornblath, D. R. (2005). Rhabdomyolysis: An evaluation of 475 hospitalized patients. Medicine, 84(6), 377-385.

Zutt, R., van der Kooi, A. J., Linthorst, G. E., Wanders, R. J., & de Visser, M. (2014). Rhabdomyolysis: Review of the literature. Neuromuscular Disorders, 24(8), 651-659. https://www.ncbi.nlm.nih.gov/pmc/articles/PMC3940504/

About The Author

Jacob McClain stands as a distinguished figure in the realm of genetic disorders research, with a career marked by unwavering dedication and groundbreaking contributions. His pioneering work has not only expanded our understanding of genetic anomalies but has also paved the way for innovative approaches in diagnosis and treatment.

Over the course of his illustrious career, Jacob McClain has demonstrated an exceptional commitment to unraveling the complexities of genetic disorders. His research endeavors have contributed significantly to identifying novel genetic markers, elucidating pathophysiological mechanisms, and advancing our knowledge in the field.

McClain's research extends beyond the laboratory, with a profound impact on clinical practices. His discoveries have played a crucial role in shaping diagnostic protocols and therapeutic interventions for individuals affected by various genetic disorders, offering hope and improved outcomes for patients worldwide.

Renowned for his collaborative spirit, McClain has spearheaded interdisciplinary efforts, bringing together experts from genetics, medicine, and related fields. Through these initiatives, he has fostered a holistic approach to understanding and addressing genetic disorders, emphasizing the importance of collaborative research in the pursuit of comprehensive solutions.

In addition to his research endeavors, McClain is a dedicated advocate for education in the field of genetic disorders. He has mentored numerous aspiring researchers, fostering the next generation of experts and instilling a passion for advancing knowledge in this critical area of healthcare.

Jacob McClain's legacy is one of profound impact and transformative contributions to the field of genetic disorders. His relentless pursuit of scientific excellence and commitment to improving patient outcomes have left an indelible mark, shaping the landscape of genetic research and clinical care.